Spiritual Veganism

Vegan Wisdom Of The Ages

Cuauhtemoc

These writings are a point of view gathered from the sayings of spiritual leaders and quotes from spiritual texts on vegan and vegetarian lifestyles, and the treatment of animals by humans. This is in no way a book to persuade anyone into a way of life or to follow any beliefs.

Cuauhtemoc

Believe Nothing.
No matter where you read it,
Or who said it,
Even if I have said it,
Unless it agrees with your own reason,
And your own common sense.
Buddha (563-483 BC)

Let no outside source but your heart feeling alone, determine your truth. You will know it when you come across truth because truth vibrates your being and feels right for you.

Cuauhtemoc

INTRODUCTION

There are many now who are turning to the vegetarian, vegan, or the raw food lifestyle. People are looking for alternative ways of healing and well being. People have tried the mainstream medical way and few have seen a positive outcome. Surgeries may remove a diseased area but leave you with missing organs and certain restrictions in your life. Medication only numbs your condition and brings numerous side effects. I went through anxiety and panic attacks and the medication gave me more anxiety, suicidal thoughts, and high states of fear and paranoia. All those side effects were written on the bottle.

The following is a study by Dr. Richard Schulze.

"The Average American"

The average American eats a low nutrition, high fat, high sugar food program, high in over processed nutritionally deplete food.

The average American drinks 300 soft drinks a year,

eats 170 pounds of white refined sugar,

eats 400 candy bars a year and

eats 500 donuts.

The average American eats 12 entire 3000 pound cows in their lifetime.

Eats 6 entire whole pigs in their entire lifetime.

Eats 3,000 chickens and/or other birds.

Eats 3,000 assorted fish and sea creatures.

Consumes 30,000 quarts of milk in their lifetime.

All of which then flows through their digestive track and their blood stream.

It's a wonder why our arteries and digestion don't work.

The average American has 2 to 4 bowel movements a week. That puts us 70,000 normal bowel movements short in our lifetime. They definitely have diverticulosis, digestive and elimination diseases.

The average American gets little exercise, has hypercholesterolemia, hypertension and high blood pressure.

The Average American consumes 30,000 aspirin and other pain killers in their lifetime. Believe me these are not people who want to feel what's going on in their body. The average American consumes 20,000 more over the counter prescription drugs and 2,000 gallons of alcohol. We are talking about someone that is very numb here or wants to numb their body.

The average American has a negative self image. The average American gets reoccurring bouts of depression and anxiety. The average American is physically, emotionally and spiritually sick and sitting in front of that tube watching more re-runs of dysfunctional television.

~

As you can see we have been numbing ourselves in these modern times. Our lifestyle is killing us and medicine isn't helping. I had to find alternative ways of healing myself when I was going through anxiety and panic. I started doing raw juice detoxes for a month at a time while taking natural herbs. I also practiced yoga with a yogi from India. Studying with this eastern man, he emphasized the breath and spiritual understanding of yoga. He taught about the energy science of the body. He taught about the vegan spiritual lifestyle. I also started learning holistic energy modalities. I learned through this journey that there was a spiritual science and veganism was part of that science.

What if we started to look back at history and observe how people lived in times of old? There are scriptures from every religion or spiritual background where there is someone who lived from 100 to 300 years of age. There is a healthy spiritual lifestyle that has been followed by many. What if we took some of that advice and followed it? What if we listened to our bodies and tried a different way of living where animals are not slaughtered? In this book I give you the vegan and vegetarian wisdom of the ages. From all spiritual traditions. Be open and accept what resonates with your being.

Cuauhtemoc

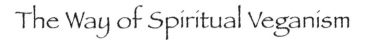
The Way of Spiritual Veganism

There are three ways of killing that we, as Buddhists, have to restrain: either by directly killing, indirectly killing, or rejoicing to see others be killed. Not only does this apply to human life, it should be also extended to all living beings.

Zen Master Thich Thanh Tu

from *Buddhism for Beginners*

One is not a great one because one defeats or harms other living beings. One is so called because one refrains from defeating or harming other living beings.

The Dhammapada

If a man can control his body and mind and thereby refrains from eating flesh and animal products, I say he will really be liberated.

The Buddha from *the Surangama Sutra*

And the flesh of slain beasts in his body will become his own tomb. For I tell you truly, he who kills, kills himself, and who so eats the flesh of slain beasts, eats of the body of death. For in his blood every drop of their blood turns to poison; in his breath their breath to stink; in his flesh their flesh to boils; in his bones their bones to chalk; in his bowels their bowels to decay; in his eyes their eyes to scales; in his ears their ears to waxy issue. And their death will become his death.

Jesus from *The Essene Gospel of Peace*

I do not regard flesh-food as necessary for us at any stage and under any clime in which it is possible for human beings ordinarily to live. I hold flesh-food to be unsuited to our species.

Mahatma Gandhi

Obey, therefore, the words of God: 'Behold, I have given you every herb bearing seed, which is upon the face of all the earth, and every tree, in the which is the fruit of a tree yielding seed; to you it shall be for meat. And to every beast of the earth, and to every fowl of the air, and to everything that creepeth upon the earth, wherein there is breath of life, I give every green herb for meat. Also the milk of every thing that moveth and liveth upon earth shall be meat for you; even as the green herb have I given unto them, so I give their milk unto you. But flesh, and the blood which quickens it, shall ye not eat.

Jesus from *The Essene Gospel of Peace*

To become vegetarian is to step into the stream which leads to nirvana.

The Buddha

And Jesus continued: "God commanded your forefathers: 'Thou shalt not kill.' But their heart was hardened and they killed. Then Moses desired that at least they should not kill men, and he suffered them to kill beasts. And then the heart of your forefathers was hardened yet more, and they killed men and beasts likewise. But I do say to you: Kill neither men, nor beasts, nor yet the food which goes into your mouth. For if you eat living food, the same will quicken you, but if you kill your food, the dead food will kill you also. For life comes only from life, and from death comes always death. For everything which kills your foods, kills your bodies also. And everything which kills your bodies kills your souls also. And your bodies become what your foods are, even as your spirits, likewise, become what your thoughts are. Therefore, eat not anything which fire, or frost, or water has destroyed. For burned, frozen and rotted foods will burn, freeze and rot your body also. Be not like the foolish husbandman who sowed in his ground cooked, and frozen, and rotten seeds. And the autumn came, and his fields bore nothing. And great was his distress. But be like that husbandman who sowed in his field living seed, and whose field bore living ears of wheat, paying a hundredfold for the seeds which he planted. For I tell you truly, live only by the fire of life, and prepare not your foods with the fire of death, which kills your foods, your bodies and your souls also."

"Master, where is the fire of life?" asked some of them.

"In you, in your blood, and in your bodies."

"And the fire of death?" asked others.

"It is the fire which blazes outside your body, which is hotter than your blood. With that fire of death you cook your foods in your homes and in your fields. I tell you truly, it is the same fire which destroys your foods and your bodies, even as the fire of malice, which ravages your thoughts, ravages your spirits. For your body is that which you eat, and your spirit is that which you think. Eat nothing, therefore, which a stronger fire than the fire of life has killed. Wherefore, prepare and eat all fruits of trees, and all grasses of the fields, and all milk of beasts good for eating. For all these are fed and ripened by the fire of life; all are the gift of the angels of our Earthly Mother. But eat nothing to which only the fire of death gives savor, for such is of Satan."

Jesus from *The Essene Gospel of Peace*

Eat not unclean foods brought from far countries, but eat always that which your trees bear. For your God knows well what is needful for you, and where and when. And he gives to all peoples of all kingdoms for food that which is best for each. Eat not as the heathen do, who stuff themselves in haste, defiling their bodies with all manner of abominations.

Jesus from *The Essene Gospel of Peace*

If you have men who will exclude any of God's creatures from the shelter of compassion and pity, you will have men who will deal likewise with their fellow men.

Francis of Assisi

By observation of the natural tendency of the organs of sense...the guideposts for determining what is nutritious...by which all animals are directed to their food, we find that when the carnivorous animal finds prey, he becomes so much delighted that his eyes begin to sparkle; he boldly seizes the prey and greedily laps the jetting blood.

On the contrary, the herbivorous animal refuses even his natural food, leaving it untouched, if it is sprinkled with a little blood. His senses of smell and sight lead him to select grasses and other herbs for his food, which he tastes with delight. Similarly with the frugivorous animals, we find that their senses always direct them to fruits of the trees and fields.

Swami Sri Yukteswar

In order to have magnetism, keep your body free from poisons. If your body is filled with poisons, your energy is more or less bound up. Raw food produces magnetism.

Too much meat causes you to lose your magnetism because animal magnetism tampers with your spiritual magnetism.

Swami Paramhansa Yogananda

So eat always from the table of God: the fruits of the trees, the grain and grasses of the field, the milk of beasts, and the honey of bees. For everything beyond these is of Satan, and leads by the way of sins and of diseases unto death. But the foods which you eat from the abundant table of God give strength and youth to your body, and you will never see diseases. For the table of God fed Methuselah of old, and I tell you truly, if you live even as he lived, then will the God of the living give you also long life upon the earth as was his.

Jesus from *The Essene Gospel of Peace*

Meat causes you to concentrate on the physical plane too much, and you tend to attract physical companions instead of spiritual ones. Meat also overstimulates sexual desire.

Swami Paramhansa Yogananda

They too, are created by the same loving hand of God which Created us...It is our duty to Protect Them and to promote their well-being.

Mother Teresa.

Are not five sparrows sold for two pennies? And not one of them is forgotten before God.

Luke 12:6

And God said, Behold, I have given you every herb bearing seed, which is upon the face of all the Earth, and every tree, in which is the fruit of a tree yielding seed; to you it shall be for meat.

Genesis 1:29-30

Man's fate is like that of the animals; the same fate awaits them both: As one dies, so dies the other. All have the same breath, man has no advantage over the animal. Everything is meaningless. All go to the same place; all come from dust and to dust all return. Who knows if the spirit of man rises upward and if the spirit of the animal goes down into the earth?

For that which befalleth the sons of men, befalleth beasts...As one dieth so dieth the other. Yet they have all one breath. So that a man hath no pre-eminence over a beast.

Ecclesiastes 3:19

A good deed done to an animal is as meritorious as a good deed done to a human being, while an act of cruelty to an animal is a bad as an act of cruelty to a human being.

Prophet Mohammed

"To what purpose is the multitude of your sacrifices unto me?" saith the LORD:

"I am full of the burnt offerings of rams, and the fat of fed beasts; and I delight not in the blood of bullocks, or of lambs, or of goats.

When ye come to appear before me, who hath required this at your hand, to tread my

courts? Bring no more vain oblations; incense is an abomination unto me; the new moons and sabbaths, the calling of assemblies, I cannot away with; it is iniquity, even the solemn meeting.

Your new moons and your appointed feasts my soul hateth: they are a trouble unto me; I am weary to bear them.

And when ye spread forth your hands, I will hide mine eyes from you: yea, when ye make many prayers, I will not hear: your hands are full of blood.

Wash you, make you clean; put away the evil of your doings from before mine eyes; cease to do evil"

Isaiah 1:11-16 (King James Version)

Alcohol benumbs the senses, deadens the reason, and inflames the baser passions and animal instincts. It is the enemy of reason, the great paralyzer of good judgement, and the destroyer of mankind.

Liquor corrodes the stomach and destroys intuition. It anesthetizes the spiritual brain cells and eventually destroys permanently their ability to tune into god consciousness. No instrument fine enough to perceive god can ever be devised--only spiritual brain cells of man can do that. It is in your own best interest to avoid alcohol. Do that which will bring you lasting happiness.

Swami Paramhansa Yogananda

And it came to pass that the Lord departed from the City and went over the mountains with his disciples. And they came to a mountain whose ways were steep and there they found a man with a beast of burden. But the horse had fallen down, for it was over laden, and he struck it till the blood flowed.

And Jesus went to him and said: "Son of cruelty, why strikest thou thy beast? Seest thou not that it is too weak for its burden, and knowest thou not that it suffers?"

But the man answered and said: "What hast thou to do therewith? I may strike it as much as it pleases me, for it is mine own, and I bought it with a goodly sum of money. Ask them who are with thee, for they are of mine acquaintance and know thereof."

And some of the disciples answered and said: "Yea, Lord, it is as he said, We have seen when he bought it.

And the Lord said again "See ye not then how it bleeds, and hear ye not also how it wails and laments ?"

But they answered and said: "Nay, Lord, we hear not that it wails and laments?"

And the Lord was sorrowful, and said: "Woe unto you because of the dullness of your hearts, ye hear not how it laments and cries unto the heavenly Creator for mercy, but thrice woe unto him against whom it cries and wails in its pain."

And he went forward and touched it, and the horse stood up, and its wounds were healed.

But to the man he said: "Go now thy way and strike it henceforth no more, if thou also desires to find mercy."

And seeing the people come unto him, Jesus, said unto his disciples, "Because of the sick I am sick; because of the hungry I am hungry; because of the thirsty I am thirsty." He also said, "I have come to end the sacrifices and feasts of blood, and if ye cease not offering and eating of flesh and blood, the wrath of God shall not cease from you, even as it came to your fathers in the wilderness, who lusted for flesh, and they ate to their content, and were filled with rottenness, and the plague consumed them."

Jesus from *The Gospel Of The Holy Twelve*

It came to pass one day as Jesus had finished his discourse, in a place near Tiberias where there are seven wells, a certain young man brought live rabbits and pigeons, that he might have to eat with his disciples.

And Jesus looked on the young man with love and said to him, "Thou hast a good heart and God shall give thee light, but knowest thou not that God in the beginning gave to man the fruits of the earth for food, and did not make him lower than the ox, or the horse, or the sheep, that he should kill and eat the flesh and blood of his fellow creatures. Ye believe that Moses indeed commanded such creatures to be slain and offered in sacrifice and eaten, as ye do in the temple, but behold a greater than Moses is here and he comes to put away the bloody sacrifices of the law, and the feasts on them, and to restore to you the pure oblation and bloodless sacrifice as in the beginning, even the grains and fruits of the earth. Of that which ye offer unto God in purity shall ye eat, but of that kind which ye offer not in purity shall ye not eat, for the hour cometh when your sacrifices and feasts of blood shall cease, and ye shall worship God with a holy worship and a pure oblation. Let these creatures therefore go free, that they may rejoice in God and bring no guilt to man."

And the young man set them free, and Jesus broke their cages and their bonds. But lo, they feared lest they should again be taken captive, and they went not away from him, but he spoke unto them and dismissed them, and they obeyed his word, and departed in gladness

Jesus *The Gospel Of The Holy Twelve*

Meat, which retains the vibrations of pain, fear, and anger of the dying animal, and denatured foods are irritating and disturbing to the equilibrium of the mind, which is thus robbed of its birthright of power to direct life energy to heal any part of the body. While food itself cannot heal, natural foods indirectly produce health by keeping the mind calm, thus permitting the life energy to flow unobstructed.

Swami Paramhansa Yogananda

Not to hurt our humble brethren is our first duty to them, but to stop there is not enough. We have a higher mission--to be of service to them wherever they require it.

Francis of Assisi

By observation of the digestive canal we find that the bowels of carnivorous animals are 3 to 5 times the length of their body, measuring from the mouth to the anus; and their stomach is almost spherical. The bowels of the herbivores are 20 to 28 times the length of their body and their stomach is more extended and of compound build. But the bowels of the frugivorous animals are 10 to 12 times the length of their body; their stomach is somewhat broader than that of the carnivorous and has a continuation in the duodenum serving the purpose of a second stomach.

This is exactly the formation we find in human beings, though Anatomy says that the human bowels are 3 to 5 times the length of man's body...making the mistake by measuring the body from crown to the soles, instead of from the mouth to anus. Thus we can again draw the inference that man is, in all probability, a frugivorous animal.

Swami Sri Yukteswar

And as Jesus was going to Jericho there met him a man with a cage full of birds which he had caught and some young doves. And he saw how they were in misery having lost their liberty, and moreover being tormented with hunger and thirst.

And he said unto the man, "What does thou do with these?"

And the man answered, "I go to make my living by selling these birds which I have taken."

And Jesus said, "What thinkest thou, if another, stronger than thou or with greater craft, were to catch thee and bind thee, or thy wife, or thy children, and cast thee into a prison, in order to sell thee into captivity for his own profit, and to make a living? Are not these thy fellow creatures, only weaker than thou? And does not the same God our Father-Mother care for them as for thee? Let these thy little brethren and sisters go forth into freedom and see that thou do this thing no more, but provide honestly for thy living."

And the man marveled at these words and at his authority, and he let the birds go free. So when the birds came forth they flew unto Jesus and stood on his shoulder and sang unto him. And the man inquired further of his doctrine, and he went his way, and learnt the craft of making baskets, and by this craft he earned his bread, and afterwards he broke his cages and his traps, and became a disciple of Jesus.

Jesus from *The Gospel Of The Holy Twelve*

And on a certain day as he was passing by a mountain side nigh unto the desert, there met him a lion and many men were pursuing him with stones and javelins to slay him.

But Jesus rebuked them, saying, "Why hunt ye these creatures of God, which are more noble than you? By the cruelties of many generations they were made the enemies of man who should have been his friends. If the power of God is shown in them, so also is shown his long suffering and compassion. Cease ye to persecute this creature who desires not to harm you, see ye not how he flees from you, and is terrified by your violence?"

And the lion came and lay at the feet of Jesus, and showed love to him; and the people were astonished, and said, "Lo, this man loves all creatures and has power to command even these beasts from the desert, and they obey him."

Jesus from *The Gospel Of The Holy Twelve*

Now if we observe the formation of the teeth in man we find that they do not resemble those of the carnivorous, neither do they resemble the teeth of the herbivorous or the omnivorous. They do resemble, exactly, those of the frugivorous animals. The reasonable inference, therefore, is that man is a frugivorous or fruit-eating animal.

Swami Sri Yukteswar

And some of his disciples came and told him of a certain Egyptian, a son of Belial, who taught that it was lawful to torment animals, if their sufferings brought any profit to men.

And Jesus said unto them, "Verily I say unto you, they who partake of benefits which are gotten by wronging one of God's creatures, cannot be righteous: nor can they touch holy things, or teach the mysteries of the kingdom, whose hands are stained with blood, or whose mouths are defiled with flesh. God gives the grains and the fruits of the earth for food, and for righteous man truly there is no other lawful sustenance for the body. The robber who breaks into the house made by man is guilty, but they who break into the house made by God, even of the least of these are the greater sinners. Wherefore I say unto all who desire to be my disciples, keep your hands from bloodshed and let no flesh meat enter your mouths, for God is just and bountiful, who ordains that man shall live by the fruits and seeds of the earth alone. But if any animal suffers greatly, and if its life be a misery unto it. or if it be dangerous to you, release it from its life quickly, and with as little pain as you can. Send it forth in love and mercy, but torment it not, and God the Father-Mother will show mercy unto you, as ye have shown mercy unto those given into your hands. And whatsoever ye do unto the cast of these my children, ye do it unto me. For I am in them and they are in me, Yea, I am in all creatures and all creatures are in me. In all their joys I rejoice, in all their afflictions I am afflicted. Wherefore I say unto you: Be ye kind one to another, and to all the creatures of God."

Jesus from *The Gospel Of The Holy Twelve*

The gods created certain kinds of beings to replenish our bodies...they are the trees and the plants and the seeds.

Plato

This hermit was Matheno, priest of Egypt, master from the temple of Sakara. When John was seven years of age Matheno took him to the wilderness and in the cave of David they abode. Matheno taught, and John was thrilled with what the master said, and day by day Matheno opened up to him the mysteries of life. John loved the wilderness; he loved his master and his simple fare. Their food was fruits, and nuts, wild honey and the carob bread. Matheno was an Isrealite, and he attended all the Jewish feasts. When John was nine years old Matheno took him to a great feast in Jerusalem. The wicked Archelaus had been deposed and exiled to a distant land because of selfishness and cruelty, and John was not afraid. John was delighted with his visit to Jerusalem. Matheno told him all about the service of the Jews; the meaning of their rites. John could not understand how sin could be forgiven by killing animals and birds and burning them before the Lord. Matheno said, The God of heaven and earth does not require sacrifice. This custom with its cruel rites was borrowed from the idol worshippers of other lands.

No sin was ever blotted out by sacrifice of animal, of bird, or man. Sin is the rushing forth of man into fens of wickedness. If one would get away from sin he must retrace his steps, and find his way out of the fens of wickedness.

The Aquarian Gospel of Jesus The Christ

The great feast of the Jews was on, and Joseph, Mary and their son, and many of their kin, went to Jerusalem. The child was ten years old. And Jesus watched the butchers kill the lambs and birds and burn them on the altar in the name of God.

His tender heart was shocked at this display of cruelty; he asked the serving priest, "What is the purpose of this slaughter of the beasts and birds? Why do you burn their flesh before the Lord?"

The priest replied, "This is our sacrifice for sin. God has commanded us to do these things, and said that in these sacrifices all our sins are blotted out."

And Jesus said, "Will you be kind enough to tell when God proclaimed that sins are blotted out by sacrifice of any kind?"

"Did not David say that God requires a sacrifice for sin? That it is a sin itself to bring before his face burnt offerings, as offerings for sin? Did not Isaiah say the same?" The priest replied, "My child you are beside yourself. Do you know more about the laws of God than all the priests of Israel? This is no place for boys to show their wit."

But Jesus heeded not his taunts; he went to Hillel, chief of the Sanhedrim, and he said to him, "Rabboni, I would like to talk with you; I am disturbed about this service of the pascal feast. I thought the temple was the house of God where love and kindness dwell. Do you not hear the bleating of those lambs, the pleading of those doves that men are killing over there? Do you not smell that awful stench that comes from burning flesh? Can man be kind and just, and still be filled with cruelty? A God that takes delight in sacrifice, in blood and burning flesh, is not my Father-God. I want to find a God of love, and you, my master, you are wise, and surely you can tell me where to find the God of love."

But Hillel could not give an answer to the child. His heart was stirred with sympathy. He called the child to him; he laid his hand upon his head and wept.

The Aquarian Gospel of Jesus The Christ

Oh, my fellow men, do not defile your bodies with sinful foods. We have corn, we have apples bending down the branches with their weight, and grapes swelling on the vines. There are sweet-flavored herbs, and vegetables which can be cooked and softened over the fire, nor are you denied milk or thyme-scented honey. The earth affords a lavish supply of riches, of innocent foods, and offers you banquets that involve no bloodshed or slaughter; only beasts satisfy their hunger with flesh, and not even all of those, because horses, cattle, and sheep live on grass.

Pythagorus

Now, Jesus with his friend Lamaas went through all the regions of Orissa, and the valley of the Ganges, seeking wisdom from the sudras and the visyas and the masters. Benares of the Ganges was a city rich in culture and in learning; here the two rabbonis tarried many days. And Jesus sought to learn the Hindu art of healing, and became the pupil of Udraka, greatest of the Hindu healers.

Udraka taught the uses of the waters, plants and earths; of heat and cold; sunshine and shade; of light and dark.

He said, "The laws of nature are the laws of health, and he who lives according to these laws is never sick. Transgression of these laws is sin, and he who sins is sick. He who obeys the laws, maintains an equilibrium in all his parts, and thus insures true harmony; and harmony is health, while discord is disease. That which produces harmony in all the parts of man is medicine, insuring health. The body is a harpsichord, and when its strings are too relaxed, or are too tense, the instrument is out of tune, the man is sick. Now, everything in nature has been made to meet the wants of man; so everything is found in medical arcanes. And when the harpsichord of man is out of tune the vast expanse of nature may be searched for remedy; there is a cure for every ailment of the flesh. Of course the will of man is remedy supreme; and by the vigorous exercise of will, man may make tense a chord that is relaxed, or may relax one that is too tense, and thus may heal himself. When man has reached the place where he has faith in God, in nature and himself, he knows the Word of power; his word is balm for every wound, is cure for all the ills of life. The healer is the man who can inspire faith. The tongue may speak to human ears, but souls are reached by souls that speak to souls. He is the forceful man whose soul is large, and who can enter into souls, inspiring hope in those who have no hope, and faith in those who have no faith in God, in nature, nor in man. There is no universal balm for those who tread the common walks of life. A thousand things produce in-harmony and make men sick; a thousand things may tune the harpsichord, and make men well. That which is medicine for one is poison for another one; so one is healed by what would kill another one. An herb may heal the one; a drink of water may restore another one; a mountain breeze may bring to life one seeming past all help; A coal of fire, or bit of earth, may cure another one; and one may wash in certain streams, or pools, and be made whole. The virtue from the hand or breath may heal a thousand more; but love is queen. Thought, reinforced by love, is God's great sovereign balm."

The Aquarian Gospel of Jesus The Christ

As long as men massacre animals, they will kill each other. Indeed, he who sows the seeds of murder and pain cannot reap joy and love.

Pythagorus

Jainism is the first religion that has made vegetarianism a fundamental necessity for transforming consciousness. And they are right. Killing just to eat makes your consciousness heavy, insensitive; and you need a very sensitive consciousness—very light, very loving, very compassionate. It is difficult for a non-vegetarian to be compassionate; and without being compassionate and loving you will be hindering your own progress.

Osho

With Lazarus and his sisters, John [the Baptist] remained for certain days. In honor of the Nazarite a feast was spread, and all the people stood about the board.

And when the chief men of the town poured out the sparkling wine and offered John a cup, he took it, held it high in air, and said, "Wine makes glad the carnal heart, and it makes sad the human soul; it plunges deep in bitterness and gall the deathless spirit of the man. I took the vow of Nazar when a child, and not a drop has ever passed my lips. And if you would make glad the coming king, then shun the cup as you would shun a deadly thing."

And then he threw the sparkling wine out in the street.

The Aquarian Gospel of Jesus The Christ

The universal God is one, yet he is more than one; all things are God; all things are one. By the sweet breaths of God all life is bound in one; so if you touch a fibre of a living thing you send a thrill from the centre to the outer bounds of life. And when you crush beneath your foot the meanest worm, you shake the throne of God, and cause the sword of right to tremble in its sheath. The bird sings out its song for men, and men vibrate in unison to help it sing. The ant constructs her home, the bee its sheltering comb, the spider weaves her web, and flowers breath to them a spirit in their sweet perfumes that gives them strength to toil. Now, men and birds and beasts and creeping things are deities, made flesh; and how dare men kill anything? 'Tis cruelty that makes the world awry. When men have learned that when they harm a living thing they harm themselves, they surely will not kill, nor cause a thing that God has made to suffer pain.

The Aquarian Gospel of Jesus The Christ

"Thou Shalt Not Kill"
Exodus 20:13 - Deuteronomy 5:17

The exact Hebrew wording of this biblical phrase is *lo tirtzack.* One of the greatest scholars of Hebrew/English linguistics (in the Twentieth Century)--Dr. Reuben Alcalay--has written in his mammoth book the Complete Hebrew /English Dictionary that "tirtzach" refers to *"any kind of killing whatsoever."* The word "*lo*," as you might suspect, means "thou shalt not."

Many Bible scholars persist with the theory that Christ ate animal flesh, obviously swayed in their opinions by personal habits. The desire to accede to prejudice and uphold existing tradition has been a human characteristic for many centuries, but truth appears now even more important as man exerts his independence in so many aspects of life.

Respected Bible scholar Rev. V.A. Holmes-Gore has researched the frequent use of the word "meat" in the New Testament Gospels. He traced its meaning to the original Greek.

His findings were first published in World Forum of Autumn, 1947. He reveals that the nineteen Gospel references to "meat" should have been more accurately translated thus:

Greek word, number of references and actual meaning:

Broma- 4 - Food

Brosis - 4 - The act of eating

Phago - 3 - To eat

Brosimos - 1 - That which is eaten

Trophe - 6 - Nourishment

Prosphagon - 1 - Anything to eat

Thus, the Authorized Version of John 21:5, .'Have ye any meat?" is incorrect. It should have been translated: "Have ye anything to eat?"

"Fish" is another frequently mistranslated word in the Bible. Its reference is often not to the form of swimming life, but to the symbol by which early Christians could identify each other. It was a secret sign, needed in times of persecution, prior to official acceptance of Christianity as a state religion.

The sign of the fish was a mystical symbol and conversational password. Its name deriving from the Greek word for fish, "ichthus" Much later it was represented an acrostic, composed of leading letters of the Greek phrase, "Iesous Christos Theou Uios Soter"-"Jesus Christ, Son of God, Saviour."

Frequent references to fish are intended as symbolic of The Christ and have nothing to do with the act of eating a dead fish. But the symbol of the fish did not meet with Roman approval. They preferred the sign of the cross, choosing to concentrate more on the death of Christ than on His brilliant life. Perhaps this is one reason only ten percent of His life record appears in the canonical scriptures. Most of His first thirty years has been omitted.

*The exact Hebrew wording of this biblical phrase is **lo tirtzack** which accurately translates as **"any kind of killing whatsoever."***

From *The Nazarene Way*

In meditation I realized a literal meaning of the word "lighter." It means more light. When you eat lighter, eat less, do a fast, or eat more raw whole foods you feel lighter. You are more light than matter. You are carrying more light. So that is why one feels more spiritual or more connected.

Cuauhtemoc

Many ask me what I felt or what changed when I became vegan.

Well first I want to go over what I released from my diet. Obviously I released any kind of animal products. I also gave up drinking anything that contained caffeine or was high in sugar. I did my best to release anything processed including bottled juices. I also released alcohol consumption of any kind.

Things I noticed within the first month was my skin cleared up and brightened up, I lost weight, and it was easier to meditate.

After that I started realizing that I would rarely get angry, I was able to control my emotions, my anxiety reduced, and my meditations kept getting more intense.

About the third to fourth month being vegan I was becoming super sensitive to peoples energy, and the energy of places. I was becoming more psychic and my energy healing became more intense according to my clients. Soon after I started having a clear connection to my guides and angels in meditation.
Overall my self control increased.

Cuauhtemoc

What you put in your hair goes into your blood stream and brain
and those chemicals are the cause of migraine headaches and certain moods and behaviors.
If it is not natural and edible,
do not put it in your hair.

Cuauhtemoc

Our skin is our biggest organ.
It absorbs anything that is put or rubbed on it.
Only use organic natural substances on your skin
for what ever you use now also enters the bloodstream and affects your system.
One of the most harmful substances people use is cosmetics,
for cosmetics have many harmful cancerous substances.

Cuauhtemoc

Self control is key in our life.
When we consume things
like soda, coffee or anything that alters the body
we tend to lose control of our thoughts and body.
Your emotions may be triggered at any moment.
It becomes hard for you to stay calm and at peace.
You lose the ability to concentrate and focus to the best of your ability.
You begin to operate in life with a hyper mind
being aware of certain behaviors but not knowing why you do them.
Your mind begins to work at 100 mph and you begin to age faster.

Cuauhtemoc

Up to 60% of *the human body is water*, the brain is composed of 70% water, and the lungs are nearly 90% water. The diet to compliment our whole body is raw foods. Fruits and vegetables carry the perfect liquids for our body. They balance the energy and liquids in our body. When our brain is well hydrated it performs better. These natural foods do not mess with the electricity in the brain and body. The fluids in our joints increase and balance causing our flexibility to increases.

Cuauhtemoc

Animals attack humans because they can sense their violence.
They can sense and sometimes smell if they consume meat
and they can sense their scattered emotions and hyper mind.
If you eat animals they start to eat you from inside.
That is what is known as disease.

One of my teachers from the East

Bibliography

Animals: Mother Teresa." *The Art of Nan Sea Love*. n.p., n.d. Web. 30 Aug. 2012.

Buddha Quotes, Quotations, and Sayings." *Buddha Quotes*. n.p., n.d. Web. 30 Aug. 2012.

Ecclesiastes (New international Version)" *Bible Gateway*. Biblica Inc., 2011. Web. 30 Aug. 2012.

ssene *Gospel of Peace*. Trans. Edmond Bordeaux Szekely. Book 1. INTERNATIONAL BIOGENIC SOCIETY, 1981. Print.

Genesis (New International Version)" Bible Gateway. Biblica Inc., 2011. Web. 30 Aug. 2012.

Gospel of The Holy Twelve." *The Nazarene Way*. Trans. Gideon Jasper Richard Ouseley, Rev. n.p., n.d. Web. 30 Aug. 2012.

Isaiah (New International Version)" Bible Gateway. Biblica Inc., 2011 Web. 30 Aug. 2012.

Luke (New International Version)" Bible Gateway. Biblica Inc., 2011. Web. 30 Aug. 2012.

chulze, Richard, Dr. *Get Well : How to Create Powerful Health*. Chapter 3. Marina Del Rey: Natural Healing Publications, 2005. Print.

The Illustrated Dhammapada; Chapter 19" *Buddhanet*. Buddha Dharma Education Association: 2012. Web. 30 Aug. 2012.

The Surangama Sutra." *Buddhanet*. Buddha Dharma Education Association: 2012. Web. 30 Aug. 2012.

Thou Shalt Not Kill." *The Nazarene Way*. n.p., n.d. Web. 30 Aug 2012.

Vegan Quotes." *Think Exist*. 2012. Web. 30 Aug. 2012.

Vegan Quotes." *Vegan Club*. Scott hughes, 2008. Web. 30 Aug. 2012.

ogananda, Paramhansa, Swami. *How to Achieve Glowing Health and Vitality: The Wisdom Of Yogananda*. Vol. 6. Nevada City, CA: Crystal Clarity, 2012. 54-55, 90. Print.

ukteswar, Sri, Swami. *The Holy Science*. Los Angeles: Self Realization Fellowship, 1990. 64-65. Print.

ukteswar, Sri, Swami. "Chapter 3 The Procedure: Sutras 9-11." *The Holy Science*. Los Angeles: Self Realization Fellowship, 1990. Print.

THE AUTHOR

"Cuauhtemoc" means "One That Has Descended Like an Eagle", commonly rendered in English as "Descending, Attacking or Diving Eagle" as in the moment when an eagle folds its wings and plummets down to strike its prey, so this is a name that implies aggressiveness and determination. It is an aztec name in the nauhtl language. Cuauhtemoc was named by his father after the last Aztec Emperor.

Cuauhtemoc began his spiritual journey in 2003 when he began to experience anxiety and panic attacks. Cuauhtemoc was in a high state of fear and panic. He looked for help in the medical field and ended up taking medications that made him feel worse. He looked for help in the religious field and was told by a priest he had something evil, which worsened his condition. Cuauhtemoc met a spiritual psychologist who saw that he wasn't even functioning anymore because of what he was told, so she opened up his mind and led him to search for his own truth. Cuauhtemoc started to read anything that had to do with spirituality. He started practicing Reiki in 2004. After Reiki, his hunger for truth led him to learn over seven more healing modalities. He studied with a yogi from India and learned the inner science part of yoga that is forgotten in the west. He became vegetarian and quit drinking alcohol in 2007. Since 2007 Cuauhtemoc began to connect more and began to download quantum inter-dimensional tools for healing.

Through his hunger for truth Cuauhtemoc now communicates with his Spiritual Guides and Angels and receives downloads of energies and attunements for people. Through the Angelic Realm, Tim received the attunements for **Cosmic Interdimensional Healing** modality which he rediscovered.

For more info go to :
www.anxietyanswer.org
www.cosmic-interdimensional-healing.com

Made in the USA
Las Vegas, NV
19 January 2023

65912242R00038